DATE DUE

3.95

W9-AKE-239

OCT 22 1973	MR 30'92	
NOV 29 1973	MR 1'93	
DEC 25 1976	DEC 18 '95	
MAR 11 1976	MAR 12 '97	
MAR 23 1976	MAR 27 '97	
FEB 14 1977	24	
JAN 20 198 DE 04 '2		
APR 13 1981		
FEB. 29 1984		
MAR. 21 1984		
AP 23 '86		
AG 24 '87		
MR 28'91		
DE 19'91		

j
612.2
M

10,751

Marr, John S.
A breath of air and a breath
    of smoke

EAU CLAIRE DISTRICT LIBRARY

A
BREATH OF AIR
AND A
BREATH OF SMOKE

BY
JOHN S. MARR, M.D.

WITH ILLUSTRATIONS BY
LYNN SWEAT

EAU CLAIRE DISTRICT LIBRARY

Published by
M. EVANS AND COMPANY, INC., New York
and distributed in association with
J. B. Lippincott Company, Philadelphia and New York

70709

For Drs. B. K. Poland and J. P. Marr

Copyright © 1971 by John S. Marr, M.D.
Illustrations copyright © 1971 by M. Evans and Company
*All rights reserved under International and Pan
American Copyright Conventions*
Library of Congress Catalog Card Number: 70-161362
Manufactured in the United States of America
9 8 7 6 5 4 3 2 1

ABOUT THIS BOOK

Dr. John Marr's new book tells you what happens inside your body every time you take A BREATH OF AIR AND A BREATH OF SMOKE. For the first time you will understand the difference between inhaling air that is fresh and standing beside a smoke-stack or smoking a cigarette.

The author of this book is someone you can trust. He is the same young medical doctor whose book about drugs—THE GOOD DRUG AND THE BAD DRUG—gave you the information you needed to make up your own mind about that subject.

Using the same technique and approach and working with the same artist, Lynn Sweat, Dr. Marr gives you as much information about your body's responses to cigarette smoke as you need to make up your own mind once again.

THE AUTHOR AND ILLUSTRATOR

JOHN MARR is a Resident in Medicine at Metropolitan Hospital in New York City, concentrating in the fields of Preventive Medicine and Public Health. His previous book for primary school children, THE GOOD DRUG AND THE BAD DRUG, has already been adopted in many schools across the country. Dr. Marr has recently joined the 200,000 doctors who have given up smoking.

LYNN SWEAT is a native Texan who lives and works in Weston, Connecticut. He has illustrated many children's books, including THE GOOD DRUG AND THE BAD DRUG and ENERGY AND INERTIA for M. Evans and Company.

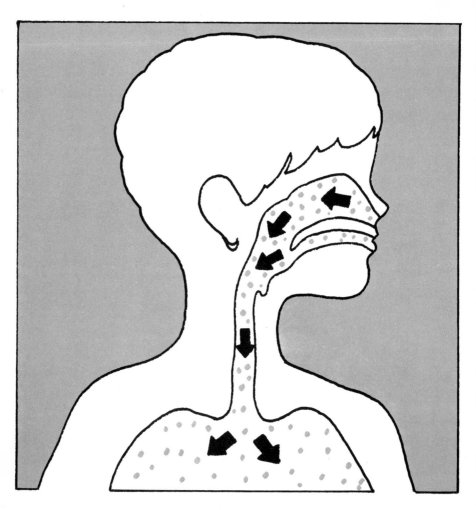

One-fifth of the air you breathe in is an odorless and colorless gas which the human body must have in order to live and grow. This gas is called oxygen. The other parts of the air you breathe in are nitrogen and a small mixture of rare gases. None of these gases is really needed by the body.

Every time you take a breath your body is both cleaning the air and removing the oxygen from it. The parts of your body that

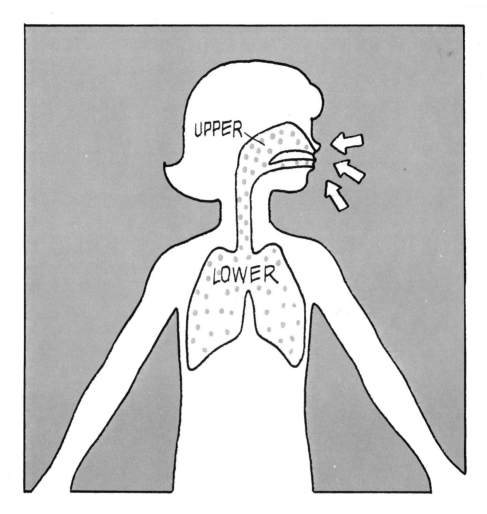

clean the air and remove the oxygen from it are called the Respiratory System. The Respiratory System has two main parts: the Upper Respiratory System and the Lower Respiratory System.

The Upper Respiratory System consists of the nose, the sinuses, and the mouth. When you breathe in air, it can go through your nose or through your mouth to your throat.

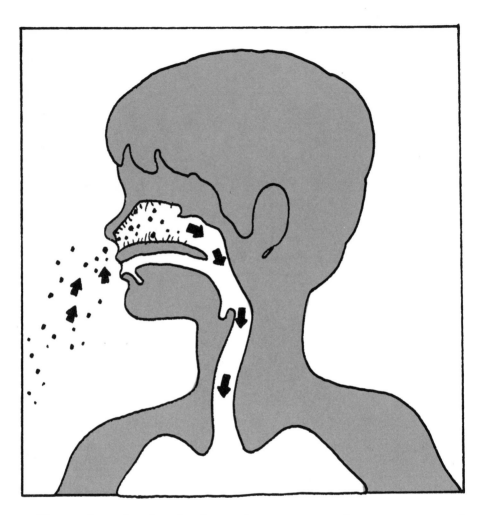

If you breathe in air through your nose, it passes up and through two nostrils. The nose helps the body breathe in air that will be clean and safe. It does this in three different ways. First, the small hairs inside your nostrils trap and filter large pieces of dirt and dust that might be in the air before they can travel farther into your body. Second, smaller pieces of dirt are trapped on the wet surfaces inside your nostrils before they travel farther into

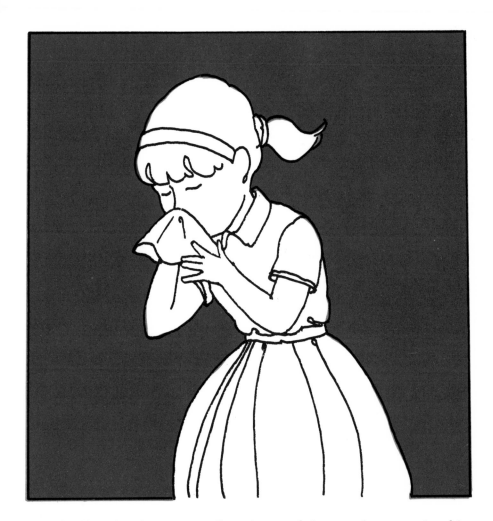

your body. Third, even smaller pieces of dust and gases mixed in the air are absorbed by special cells inside your nose. These cells are connected to your brain by nerves. They can sense odors and can warn you if the air smells bad or if food is spoiled. If there is too much dust in the air or if you are allergic to dust or pollen, these nerves make you sneeze in an attempt to keep the dust from getting inside your body.

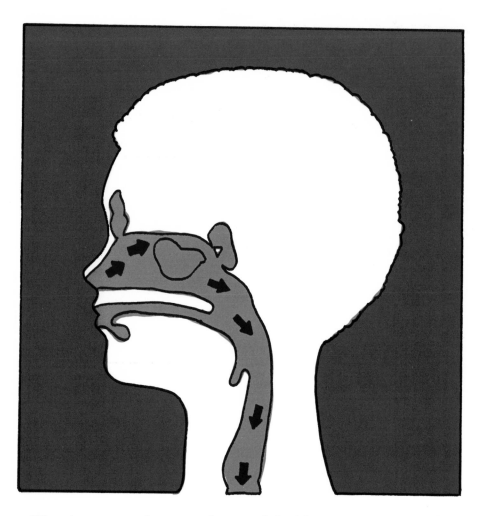

The sinuses are the second part of the Upper Respiratory System. Sinus is another name for a hollow space. There are eight sinuses in the skull. These eight hollow spaces in the bone are like little rooms where air can wait before passing into the throat.

The sinuses have three purposes. First, they make the head lighter in weight so that you can move it more easily. Second, when air is breathed in through the nostrils some of it passes into

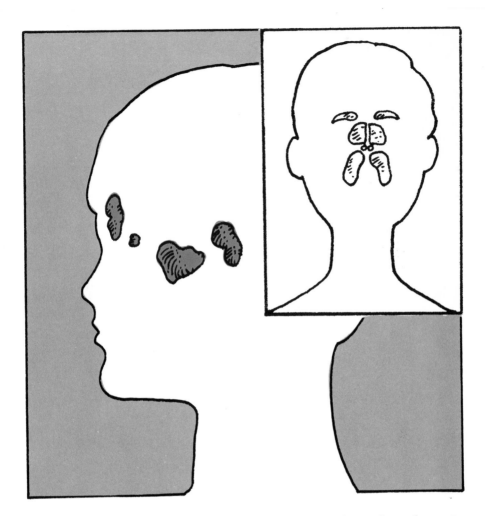

the sinuses. There, the air can be warmed gently and made moist before it enters the Lower Respiratory System. Air that has not been warmed or moistened may harm or dry out the throat and Lower Respiratory System. The third purpose of the sinuses is to help clean the air even more before it passes farther into the body.

The cells inside your nose and sinuses make a liquid called

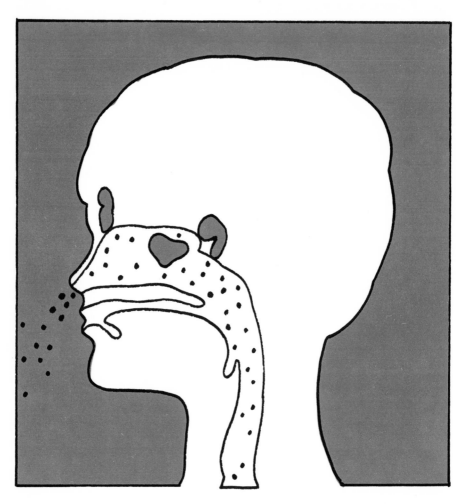

mucus. It is mucus that traps dirt, dust, and even smells. It is mucus that helps warm the air inside the sinuses and keep it moist. Sometimes too much mucus is made and your nose may run or become stopped up. This usually happens when you have a cold or when you are allergic to something. If you then breathe in air through your mouth, your throat may become dry and sore and it may become difficult to swallow. The air may make your larynx

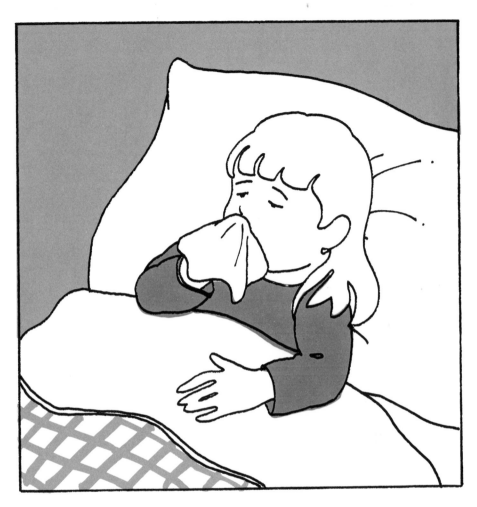

(or voice box) dry and sore and you may become hoarse. This happens because the air that is breathed in through your mouth passes directly into the Lower Respiratory System without being cleaned, warmed, and moistened by your nose and sinuses.

The Lower Respiratory System consists of the trachea (or windpipe), the bronchial tubes, and tiny balloon-like sacs called alveoli (AL-VEE-OH-LIE). The trachea is a large hollow tube that

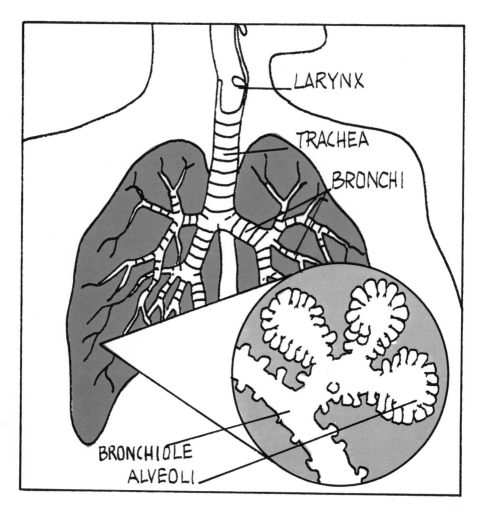

LARYNX

TRACHEA

BRONCHI

BRONCHIOLE
ALVEOLI

begins just below the larynx. It passes into the chest where it divides into two smaller tubes called bronchi (BRON-KEE). Each of these divides into two smaller bronchi, which in turn divide into even smaller bronchi. This continues twenty-three times on each side until there are millions of very small tubes spread out through the chest. This series of divisions is called the tracheo-bronchial tree (TRAY-KEE-OH-BRON-KEE-AL) because it looks like

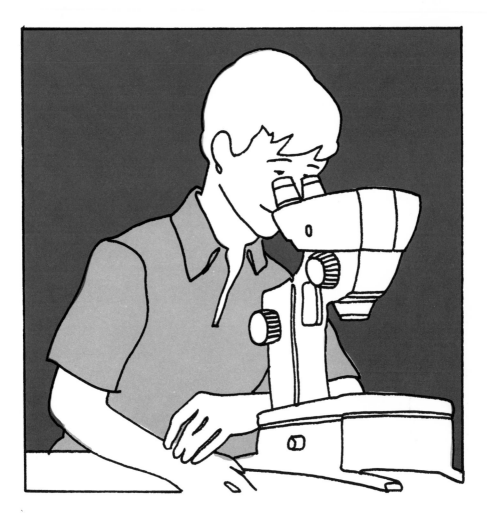

the branching of a tree upside down with the trachea being the main trunk. The smallest tube at the end of the tracheo-bronchial tree is called a bronchiole (BRON-KEE-OL). It is so small that you would need a powerful microscope to see it.

Each bronchus and bronchiole is made up of cells that are fitted together like bricks in a wall. The cells on the outside of the bronchiole support the tube and help to keep it open. Muscle cells

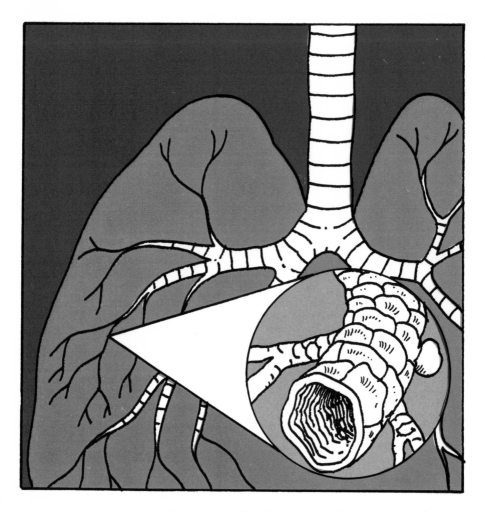

are wrapped around these small tubes also. They can help the bronchiole keep open or, if the muscle cells are irritated and tighten—the bronchiole will become narrow. If the muscle tightens too much or too long, air cannot pass through the narrow tubes. People with asthma have trouble with these muscles. When the muscles are irritated by certain dusts or pollens in the air, they contract, and breathing becomes difficult. The wheezing noise

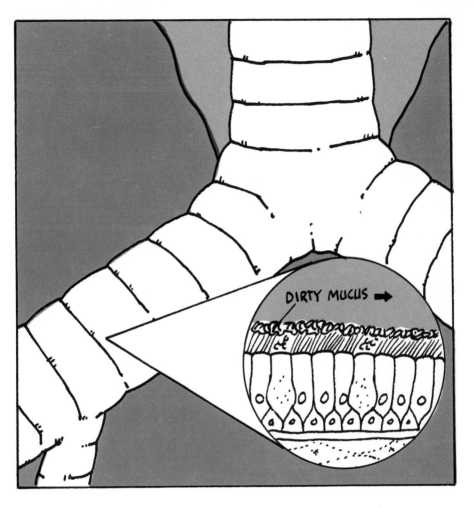

that happens during an asthma attack is the sound of air squeezing past the narrow, dry bronchioles.

The inside of the bronchiole is composed of two types of cells. One type of cell is the same kind that makes mucus in the nose and sinuses. It is called a goblet cell because it looks like a glass filled with fluid. These goblet cells make mucus that moistens the Lower Respiratory System and prevents it from drying out. The

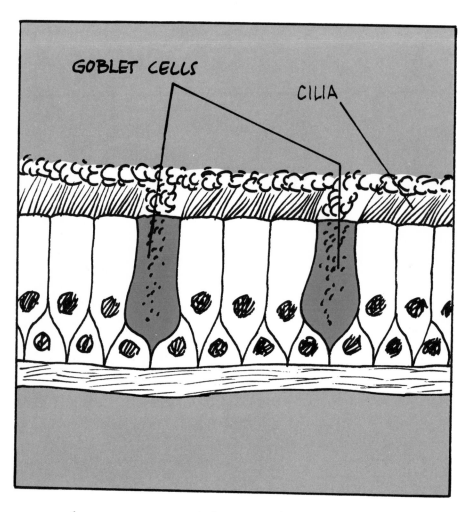

GOBLET CELLS

CILIA

mucus also traps any remaining soot, dust, and dirt that was not stopped by the Upper Respiratory System.

The second type of cell that lines the inside of the bronchiole is special. It has hundreds of tiny hairs, called cilia (SILL-EE-AH) that beat back and forth in rhythm. These tiny cilia are on every cell. Together they act like billions of small fingers passing mucus, dust, old cells, and even germs over them as if they were carry-

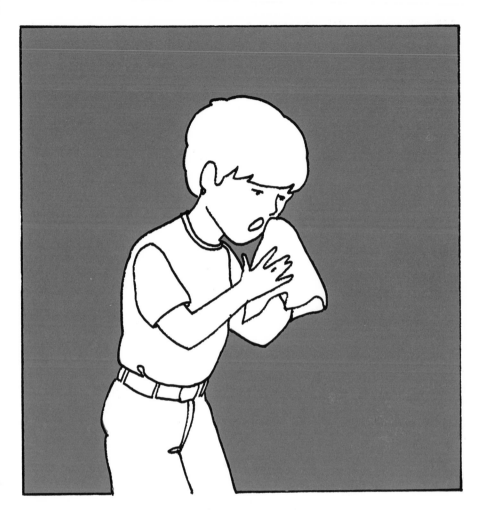

ing them. The cilia beat together slowly and surely in one direction. They gradually collect mucus with dust and germs on them and carry it up toward the trachea. The mixture is carried up through the bronchioles to the larger and larger bronchi until it arrives in the trachea. If a person coughs, he can bring the mucus up into the mouth where it can be expelled from the body. The cells of the bronchioles that produce mucus and have cilia on

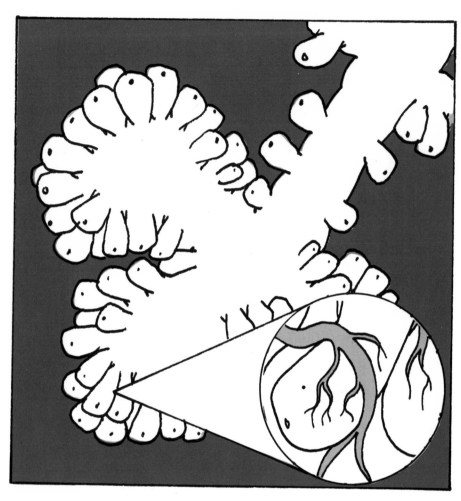

them are one of the last barriers in the Respiratory System against dirty or unclean air.

The third part of the Lower Respiratory System is the alveoli. Alveoli are tiny balloon-like sacs that open into the smallest bronchioles. There are millions of alveoli, looking like microscopic bunches of grapes attached to the stems of tiny bronchioles. All the alveoli taken together are called the lungs. So the lungs are

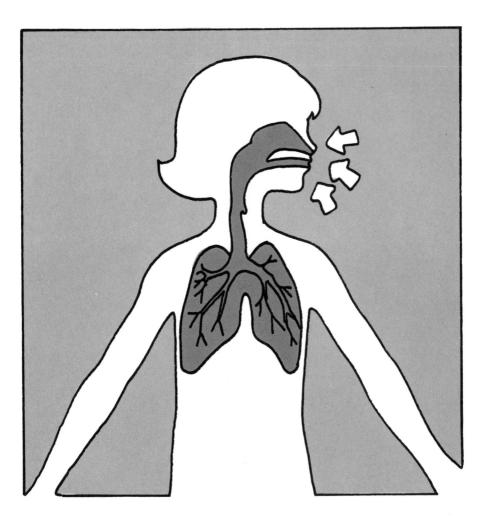

really made up of millions of tiny balloons that collect the air that is breathed in through the tracheo-bronchial tree.

When you breathe in air it passes through your mouth, or nose and sinuses, past the larynx into the trachea. Then the air passes into the bronchi, then into every bronchiole and finally into the alveoli. The oxygen in the air is then absorbed into the cells of the alveoli. The oxygen becomes part of the cells of the alveoli

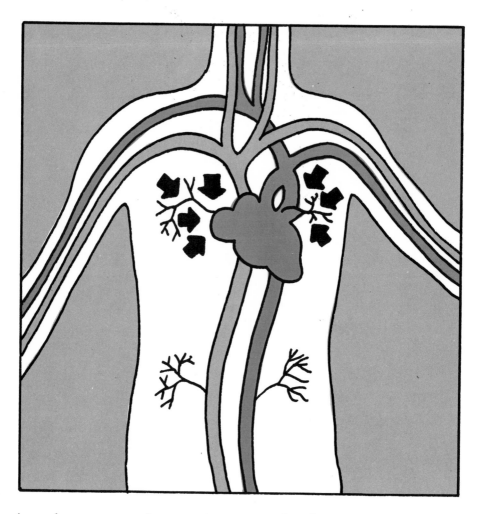

in order to get ready to go into your circulation.

Circulation is a word that describes how your blood travels throughout your body. When the oxygen crosses from the cells of your alveoli into your circulation, it becomes mixed with your blood. Your circulation (or bloodstream) depends on three parts which are connected to one another: your heart which acts like a pump; your arteries which act like pipes carrying blood away

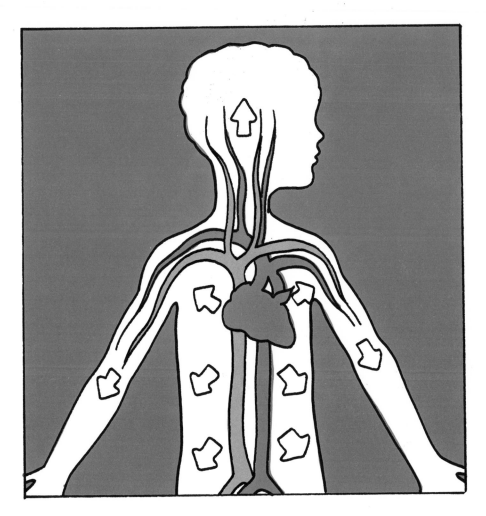

from your heart when it pumps; and your veins which act like
pipes carrying blood from the distant parts of your body to your
heart.

Once the oxygen goes through the cells of the alveoli, it is
picked up by the lung veins. When the oxygen combines with the
blood, the blood becomes rich in oxygen. Blood that is rich in
oxygen is bright red. It is then pumped back in the large lung

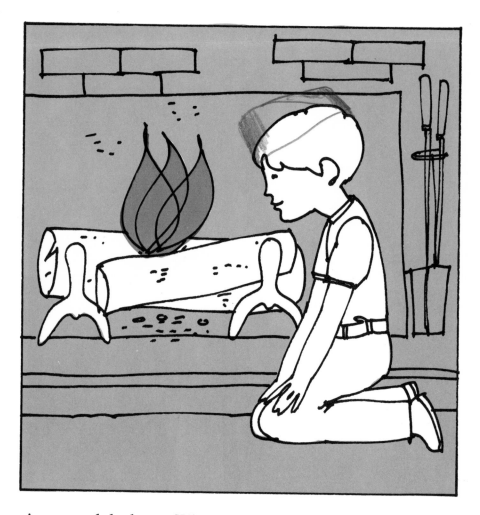

veins toward the heart. When the bright red blood arrives at the heart, it is pumped out through the heart into the arteries. These arteries carry the blood combined with oxygen to every part of your body where it is used to help make energy.

The body uses oxygen in a way similar to what happens when wood burns. Wood would not burn without oxygen. Oxygen helps it burn and helps it produce energy in the forms of fire and heat.

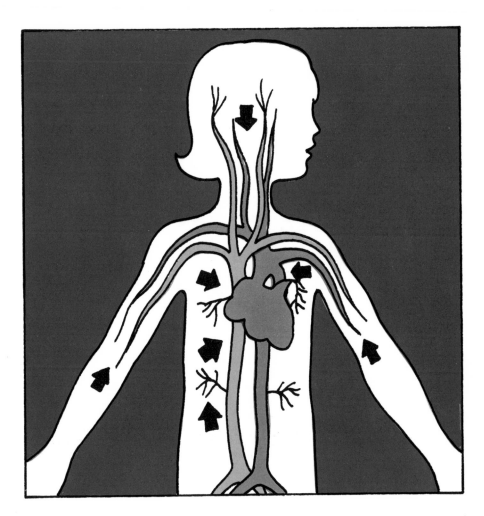

And just as there are waste gases and smoke when wood is burned to make energy, the body also produces waste gases when its own energy is being made. One of these waste gases is called carbon dioxide. The body removes this gas from the circulation, just as a fireplace sends smoke up through its chimney.

The carbon dioxide leaves the cells in all parts of your body and enters the veins. The blood in these veins is not bright red

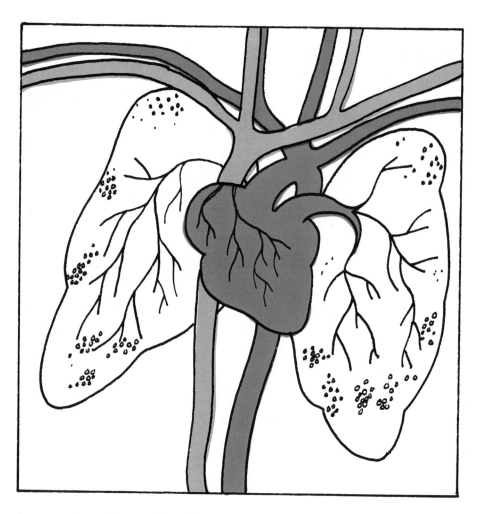

because it no longer has the oxygen in it which has been used up by the cells to make energy. The blood in veins is blue in color when there is little oxygen in it. This blood, rich in carbon dioxide but poor in oxygen, is carried by hundreds of veins toward your heart. This blood arrives at your heart and is pumped to your lungs. When the blood reaches the lung veins, oxygen from the alveoli can again combine with it while the carbon dioxide car-

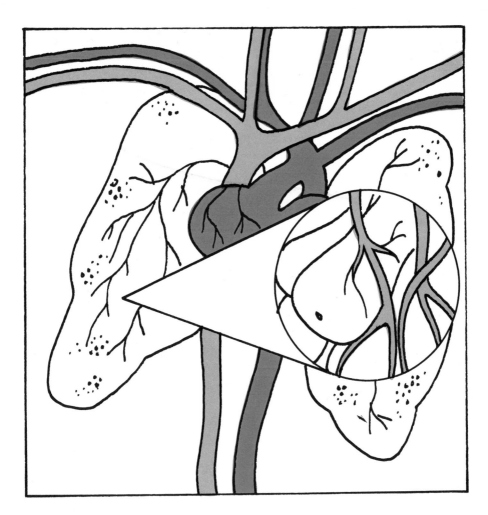

ried from the distant parts of your body passes from the lung veins into the alveoli. There carbon dioxide can be breathed out and exchanged for oxygen in the air with each breath. Thus the Respiratory System's purpose is to collect clean air and remove the oxygen from it for the body to use and at the same time rid the body of waste products, like carbon dioxide formed when the body produces energy.

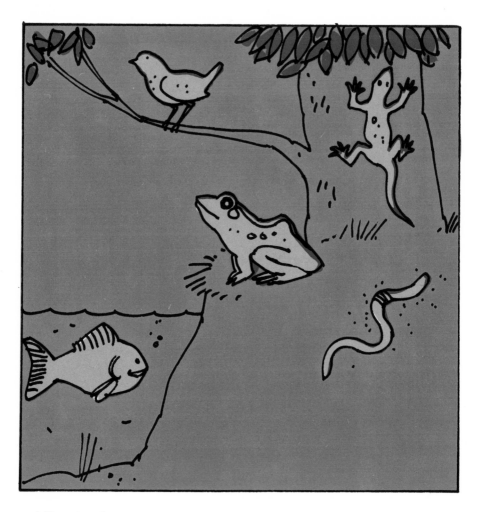

All animals use oxygen to make energy. Some have lungs to collect the oxygen; others use gills and others can even use their skins to collect the oxygen. Carbon dioxide is removed as a waste product of respiration in all animals. Plants, however, need carbon dioxide to make energy. Plants absorb carbon dioxide from the air and when they make their energy, oxygen is the waste product. The reason the air we breathe always has oxygen in it

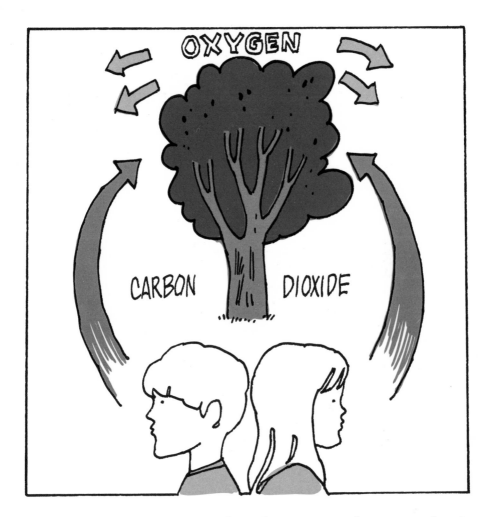

is that trees and grass and other plants renew the oxygen in air while using up the carbon dioxide.

So each time we take a breath of air—and we take almost one thousand breaths every hour—we are performing a complicated task that involves both our inside and outside environments.

Suppose the air you breathe is full of smoke. What would happen then?

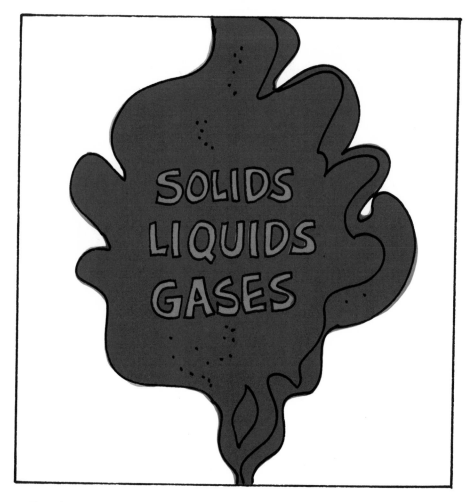

Smoke is a mixture of solids, liquids, and gases. It is formed when coal, wood, or tobacco is burned. The solid parts of smoke are small pieces of soot and ashes carried into the air. The liquid parts of smoke are called tars. The gases that are part of smoke depend on what is being burned.

When a cigarette is burned, tobacco combines with the oxygen in the air to create energy in the form of heat. Smoke is formed

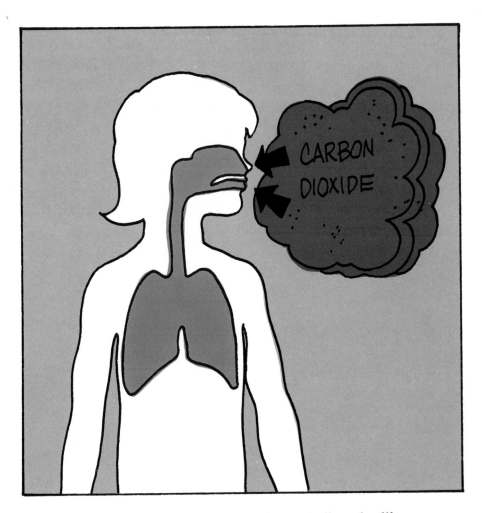

as a waste product of a cigarette when it is "smoked."

Smoke from cigarettes contains many different gases. One of these gases is carbon dioxide. The carbon dioxide in smoke is breathed in if you inhale the smoke. It cannot be used by the body to make energy. The body is actually trying to get rid of its own carbon dioxide that was formed when energy was made by its cells. If a person breathes in too much carbon dioxide, less oxy-

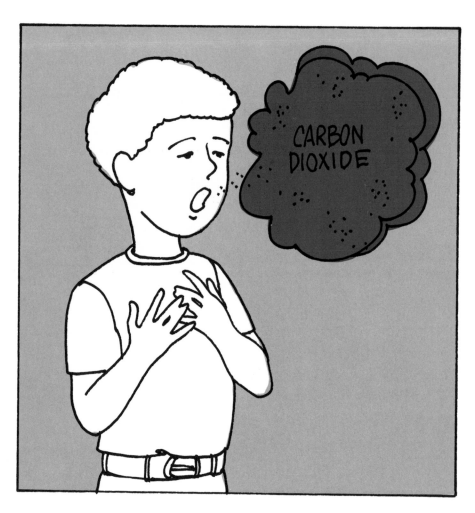

gen will be able to get into his lungs and less energy can be made. The person breathes harder and faster to get more oxygen. A person who has too much carbon dioxide in his lungs and too little oxygen will be short of breath. If less and less oxygen is breathed in and more carbon dioxide were to be inhaled until all the air in the lungs was carbon dioxide, the person would suffocate.

Another gas that is part of cigarette smoke is carbon monox-

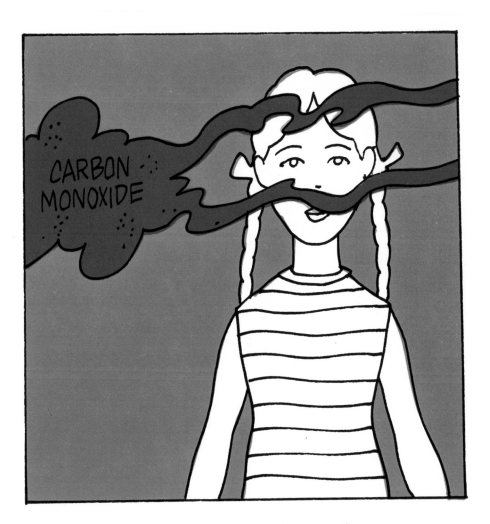

ide. In large amounts this gas can be very dangerous to your body. This is the same gas that passes through the exhaust pipe of an automobile. You cannot see, smell, or taste it. It does not irritate your eyes, nose, or tracheo-bronchial tree. You cannot tell how much of it you have breathed in. When you inhale cigarette smoke, a small part of the smoke is carbon monoxide. It passes down through your bronchioles and into your alveoli. The carbon

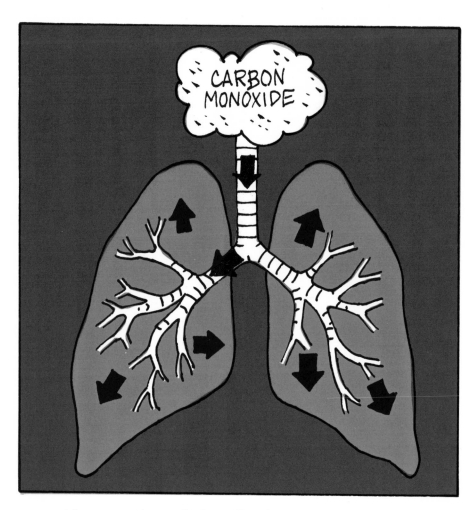

monoxide passes through the cells of the alveoli into the circulation. Carbon monoxide can combine with your blood just as oxygen does. As a result, some of the blood that leaves the lungs will not have oxygen combined with it. This blood will be carried back to the heart and out through arteries to every part of your body. Since the cells of your body can use only oxygen to make energy, this blood combined with carbon monoxide will not be used to

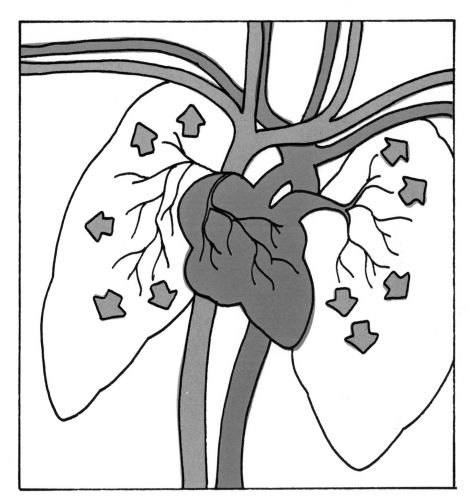

make energy. It passes unchanged back into the veins and is carried back toward the heart. It is pumped by the heart to the lungs. Unlike carbon dioxide that can be exchanged for oxygen in the lungs, carbon monoxide remains attached to the blood, making that portion of blood useless until it is slowly removed by the body, or new blood cells replace the useless ones.

People who smoke a lot usually have more carbon monoxide

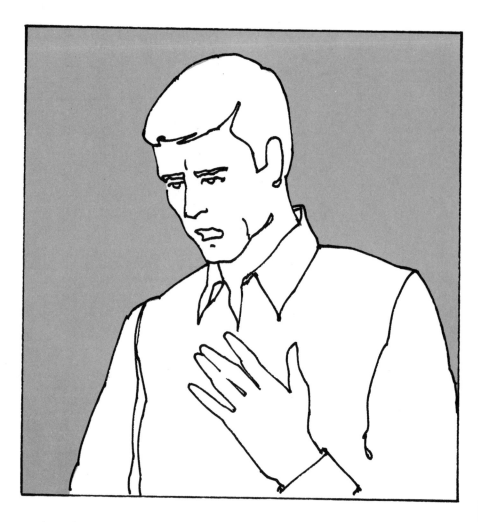

in their blood than people who do not smoke. If there is too much carbon monoxide in their blood, these people will be short of breath because they cannot breathe in enough oxygen. If these people were to stop smoking, the blood that combined with the carbon monoxide would slowly be replaced by fresh blood that would then be able to carry oxygen.

There are more than forty other gases in cigarette smoke. Some

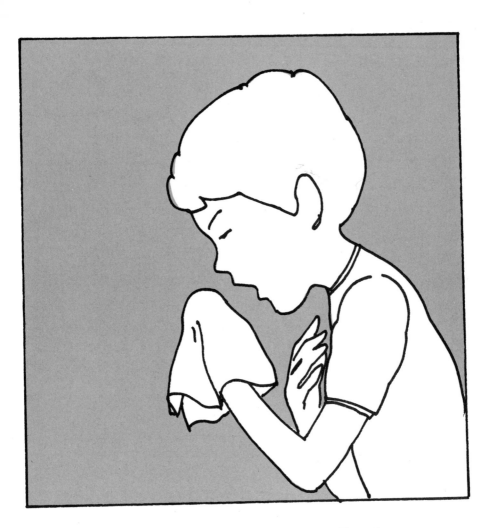

of these gases irritate the Upper and Lower Respiratory tracts. In the nose they trigger sneezing and in the trachea they trigger coughing—two reflexes the body uses to warn you that you have breathed in something harmful.

These gases also irritate the cells in the tracheo-bronchial tree. The goblet cells will produce too much mucus in an attempt to bathe the irritated cells. The gases also paralyze the cilia in the

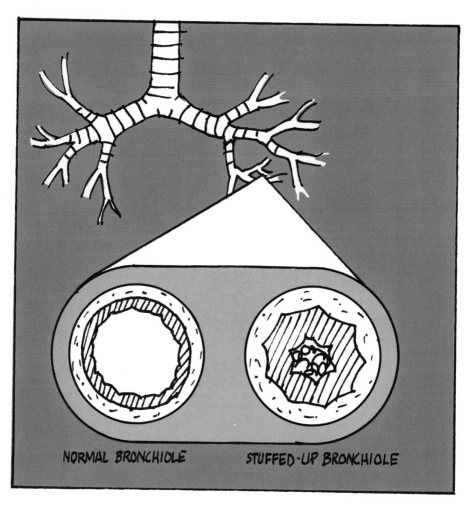

NORMAL BRONCHIOLE

STUFFED-UP BRONCHIOLE

bronchioles. When the cilia stop beating, dirt and germs can collect in the bronchioles. The cilia stop carrying excess mucus out of the bronchioles and they get stuffed up. Less air can get through. Since the cleansing system of the Lower Respiratory System is not working, infection becomes more likely.

An irritation of the bronchi and the bronchioles is called bronchitis (BRON-KITE-ISS). Bronchitis is a disease that causes fever,

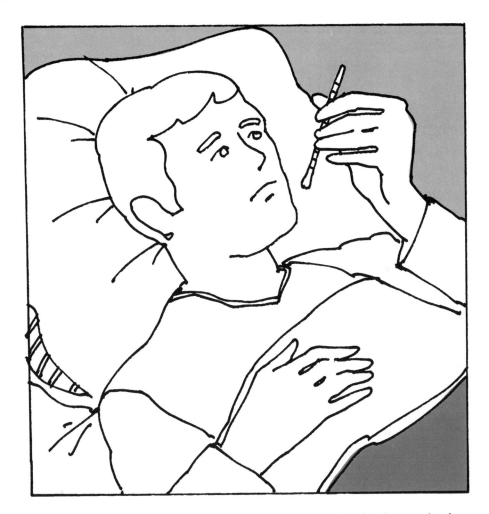

sweating, shortness of breath, weakness, and a bad cough that brings up old mucus from the stuffed-up bronchioles. Bronchitis can be caused by germs alone, but the most common cause for long-standing bronchitis is cigarette smoking.

When people with long-standing bronchitis stop smoking, their bodies slowly replace the damaged goblet cells and the cells with the cilia and the cleansing system of the Lower Respiratory Sys-

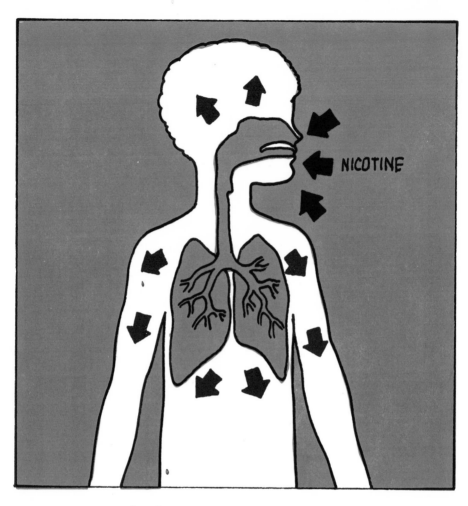

NICOTINE

tem starts to work, cleaning out germs and dirt, all over again.

Another part of cigarette smoke is nicotine. Nicotine can be a gas if it is heated. If it is cooled it becomes a liquid. In tobacco nicotine exists as tiny particles of moisture. Nicotine is a powerful drug that is turned from moisture in the tobacco into a gas by the heat of the cigarette. Nicotine travels into your Respiratory System in the same way as the other gases. The drug enters the

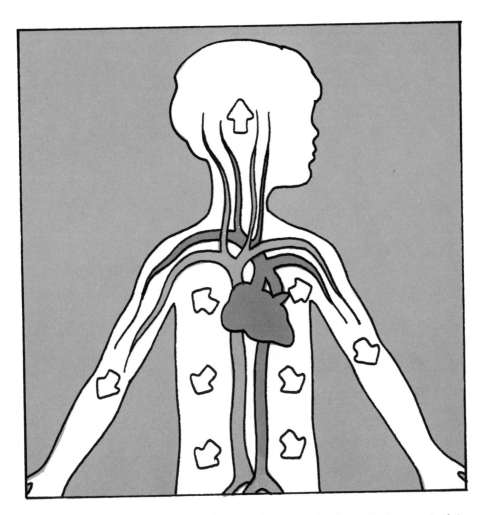

alveoli where it is absorbed into the circulation. It is carried in the blood from your lungs to your heart, then pumped out through arteries to every part of your body.

Even in very small amounts, nicotine causes the arteries in certain parts of your body to contract. Less blood is able to pass through the arteries and less oxygen can reach the distant parts of the body. The heart beats harder and faster in an attempt to

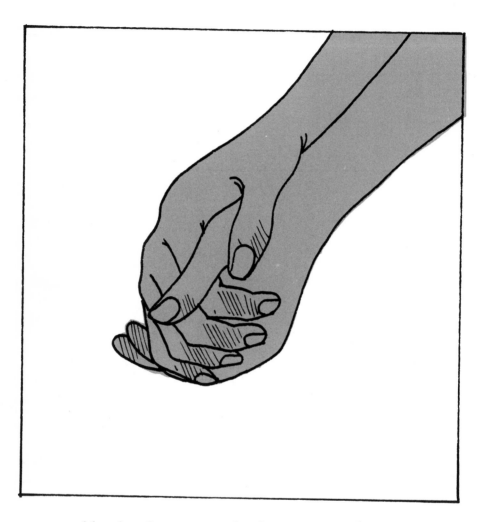

get more blood and oxygen to the distant parts of the body. People who smoke a lot usually have cold hands because the arteries of the hands are constricted and less warm blood can reach them. If there is only a little oxygen in the arteries of the hand, the hand will also turn blue.

If too much nicotine is absorbed into the circulation, it can make a person dizzy, nervous, and sick to his stomach. Nicotine

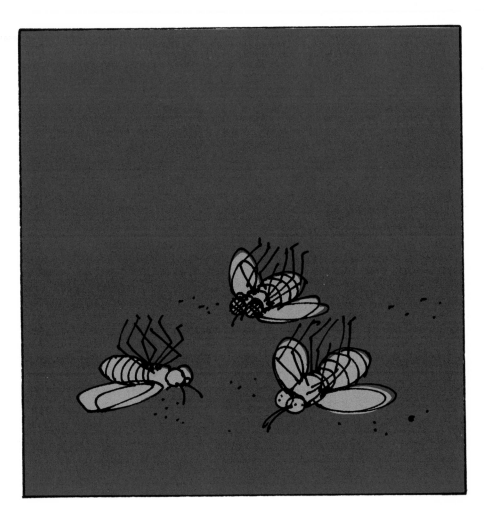

is so powerful that some people even use large doses of it as bug killer.

People who continue to smoke will slowly get used to the bad effects of nicotine. The nicotine has become a drug that is needed by the body like a normal body needs food. It peps the body up for a short time but if the body does not have a continual supply it will become uncomfortable. People who smoke cigarettes can

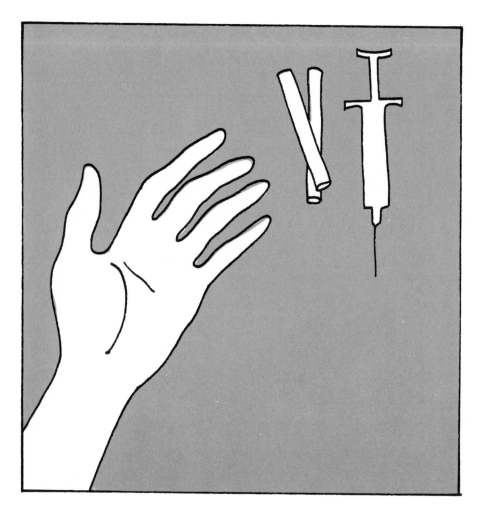

become addicted to them just as a person can get addicted to a bad drug. Many people who smoke wish they could stop smoking. However, they are addicts to the nicotine in the cigarette smoke. They are afraid of the nervousness and sick feelings they might get if they stopped smoking.

Tars are another liquid part of smoke. Tars are a mixture of thousands of complex chemicals. They are brownish in color, bit-

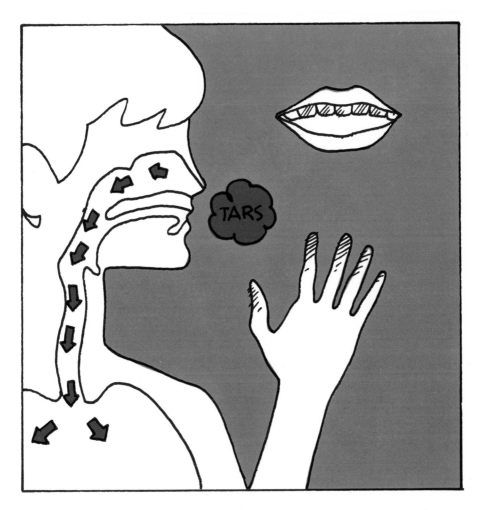

ter to taste, and sticky to touch. This is the part of the tobacco that stains the teeth and fingers of a smoker. When a cigarette is lit, the tars are turned from liquid to vapor just as water is turned into steam when it is heated in a kettle on the stove. The vaporized tars can pass through the cigarette and filter and into the Respiratory System. Tars collect on the cells of the tracheobronchial tree where they can do damage. Over a period of many

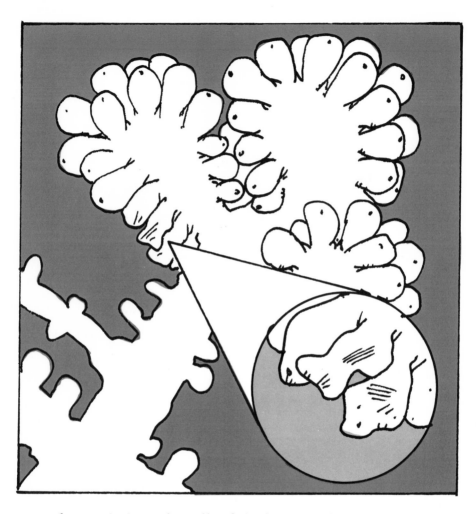

years the tars irritate the cells of the bronchioles and alveoli. Scientists still do not know which chemicals in tars cause damage, or exactly how the damage occurs. They believe that some of the tars harm the alveoli in a special way: the alveoli all over the lungs are broken up and change from elastic balloons into wrinkled and flabby sacs. Some of the alveoli collapse completely while others burst. For every air sac that bursts, less oxygen is able to

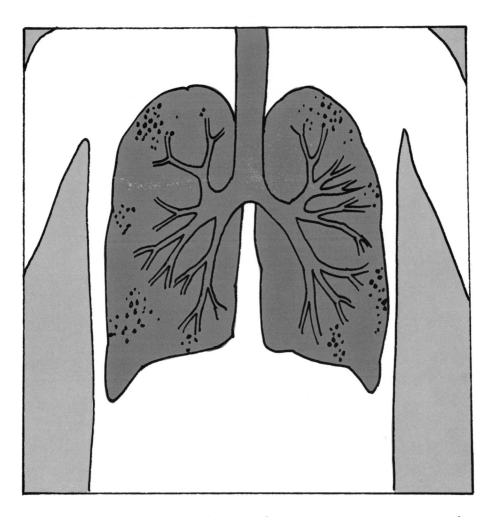

be absorbed into the circulation. If a person were to stop smoking, tars would no longer be able to irritate and damage the alveoli. However, unlike the other parts of the Respiratory System that are hurt by cigarette smoke, the alveoli cannot be replaced by the body even if a person stops smoking.

The worst diseases caused by smoking are cancer and heart disease. No one knows what part of cigarette smoke causes these

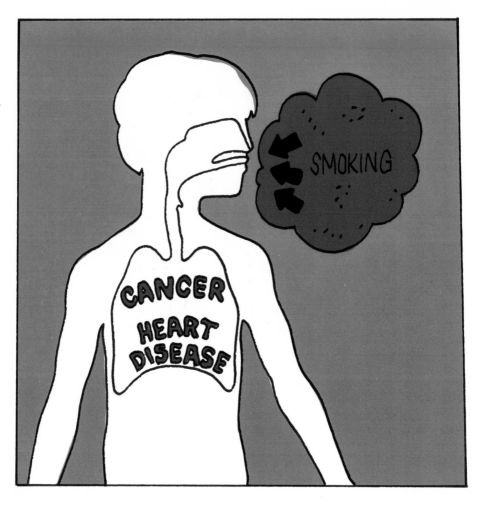

diseases. It may be a solid, a liquid, or a gas. But even though no one knows how cigarette smoking causes these diseases, certain facts are definitely known. One fact is that people who smoke a lot are ten times more likely to die from cancer of the lung and twice as likely to die from heart disease as people who do not smoke. People who smoke a lot are also more likely to get cancer in other parts of their bodies than people who don't smoke. An-

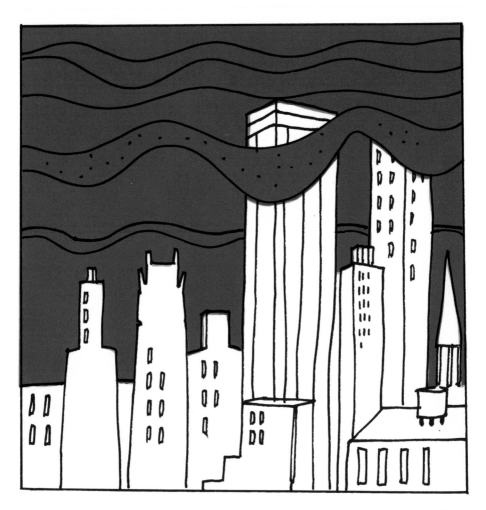

other fact is that if a person stops smoking the chances get less and less that he will get cancer or heart disease.

Scientists say that some of our air is so dirty that breathing it for one day is just as bad as smoking a pack of cigarettes. So if you also smoked a pack a day, it would be like smoking *two* packs a day.

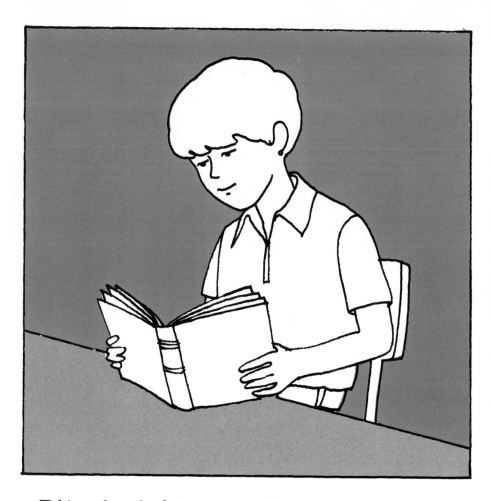

Taking a breath of air appears to be a simple thing that can be done without thinking. However there are many things that happen silently during that breath—all to insure that the body has clean air and oxygen to help make energy for work and play.

Taking a breath of smoke also appears to be a simple thing that is done without thinking. However there are many silent changes going on inside the body. If the body cannot protect itself any longer from the smoke, sickness in one form or another occurs.